Homemade Healing Salves

30 Natural Holistic Recipes

Table of Contents

Introduction

There you are, standing in line in another CVS pharmacy, looking for some sort of ointment that will help.

But help what?

It seems that this week you are dealing with dry skin, next week it's going to be a

burn, the week after that perhaps you have to deal with callouses, then you have a scrape or a scratch.

It seems that no matter what you get, you will be back in a while to find another. If only there was a remedy that you could use for more than one purpose. If only there was an all natural solution to what you are facing.

If only there was a way you could make it yourself.

Well now, there is.

And this book is the secret to learning how to do it. I want to show you just how easy it is for you to make your own healing salves, so you have what you need on hand, no matter what it is. Whether you are dealing with scrapes or burns, dry skin or callouses, I want to give you the remedy.

Using simple ingredients, you can find the solution to your problems. Simply use your favorite combinations, and you will find your dry skin disappear, your callouses soften, and never fear scars or infections again.

With the salves you find in this book, you will have the answers to all your issues, without worry that you'll have to buy something else.

Let me give you the secret to soft, beautiful skin... and get started making your own.

There's no end to the solutions you will find in this book, changing the way you view any kind of skin care product.

Are you ready?

The results are incredible.

Chapter 1 – Soft and Soothing Salves

Soothsayer Salve

What you will need:

8 drops tea tree oil

1/3 teaspoon crushed rosemary leaves

2 drops garlic oil

1/3 cup beeswax

½ cup coconut oil

¼ cup shea butter

1/3 cup sweet almond oil

Directions:

Shave the beeswax into a pan on the stove and turn on to medium heat. Add in the coconut oil, and stir as the combination melts.

Continue to stir and keep an eye on the mix, and once it's completely smooth, cut the shea butter into smaller pieces and add that as well. Once the mix is smooth once more, add in the rest of the ingredients.

Remove from heat, and let cool, stirring occasionally. You may need to use your electric mixer to keep it light and fluffy, or by just using your spoon. Transfer to another glass jar, and let finish cooling.

Store in this glass jar with an airtight lid, and keep for up to 6 months.

The Band Aid Banisher

What you will need:

8 drops tea tree oil

8 drops myrrh oil

1/3 teaspoon crushed mint leaves

1/3 cup beeswax

½ cup coconut oil

¼ cup shea butter

1/3 cup sweet almond oil

Directions:

Shave the beeswax into a pan on the stove and turn on to medium heat. Add in the coconut oil, and stir as the combination melts.

Continue to stir and keep an eye on the mix, and once it's completely smooth, cut

the shea butter into smaller pieces and add that as well. Once the mix is smooth once more, add in the rest of the ingredients.

Remove from heat, and let cool, stirring occasionally. You may need to use your electric mixer to keep it light and fluffy, or by just using your spoon. Transfer to another glass jar, and let finish cooling.

Store in this glass jar with an airtight lid, and keep for up to 6 months.

Your Best Friend

What you will need:

12 drops geranium oil

4 drops aloe

1/3 cup beeswax

½ cup coconut oil

¼ cup shea butter

1/3 cup sweet almond oil

Directions:

Shave the beeswax into a pan on the stove and turn on to medium heat. Add in the coconut oil, and stir as the combination melts.

Continue to stir and keep an eye on the mix, and once it's completely smooth, cut the shea butter into smaller pieces and add that as well. Once the mix is smooth once more, add in the rest of the ingredients.

Remove from heat, and let cool, stirring occasionally. You may need to use your electric mixer to keep it light and fluffy, or by just using your spoon. Transfer to another glass jar, and let finish cooling.

Store in this glass jar with an airtight lid, and keep for up to 6 months.

The Ultimate Cleanser
What you will need:

8 drops cinnamon oil

8 drops geranium oil

1 teaspoon aloe vera gel

1/3 cup beeswax

½ cup coconut oil

¼ cup shea butter

1/3 cup sweet almond oil

Directions:

Shave the beeswax into a pan on the stove and turn on to medium heat. Add in the coconut oil, and stir as the combination melts.

Continue to stir and keep an eye on the mix, and once it's completely smooth, cut the shea butter into smaller pieces and add that as well. Once the mix is smooth once more, add in the rest of the ingredients.

Remove from heat, and let cool, stirring occasionally. You may need to use your electric mixer to keep it light and fluffy, or by just using your spoon. Transfer to another glass jar, and let finish cooling.

Store in this glass jar with an airtight lid, and keep for up to 6 months.

The Infection Fighter Deluxe
What you will need:

½ teaspoon witch hazel

5 drops myrrh oil

1/3 cup beeswax

½ cup coconut oil

¼ cup shea butter

1/3 cup sweet almond oil

Directions:

Shave the beeswax into a pan on the stove and turn on to medium heat. Add in the coconut oil, and stir as the combination melts.

Continue to stir and keep an eye on the mix, and once it's completely smooth, cut the shea butter into smaller pieces and add that as well. Once the mix is smooth once more, add in the rest of the ingredients.

Remove from heat, and let cool, stirring occasionally. You may need to use your electric mixer to keep it light and fluffy, or by just using your spoon. Transfer to another glass jar, and let finish cooling.

Store in this glass jar with an airtight lid, and keep for up to 6 months.

Chapter 2 – A Salve and a Half

Burn be Gone
What you will need:

1 teaspoon aloe vera gel

12 drops rose oil

1 teaspoon rosemary leaves, crushed

1/3 cup beeswax

½ cup coconut oil

¼ cup shea butter

1/3 cup sweet almond oil

Directions:

Shave the beeswax into a pan on the stove and turn on to medium heat. Add in the coconut oil, and stir as the combination melts.

Continue to stir and keep an eye on the mix, and once it's completely smooth, cut the shea butter into smaller pieces and add that as well. Once the mix is smooth once more, add in the rest of the ingredients.

Remove from heat, and let cool, stirring occasionally. You may need to use your electric mixer to keep it light and fluffy, or by just using your spoon. Transfer to another glass jar, and let finish cooling.

Store in this glass jar with an airtight lid, and keep for up to 6 months.

Ups and Downs
What you will need:

1 teaspoon honey

1 teaspoon aloe vera gel

½ teaspoon witch hazel

1/3 cup beeswax

½ cup coconut oil

¼ cup shea butter

1/3 cup sweet almond oil

Directions:

Shave the beeswax into a pan on the stove and turn on to medium heat. Add in the coconut oil, and stir as the combination melts.

Continue to stir and keep an eye on the mix, and once it's completely smooth, cut the shea butter into smaller pieces and add that as well. Once the mix is smooth once more, add in the rest of the ingredients.

Remove from heat, and let cool, stirring occasionally. You may need to use your electric mixer to keep it light and fluffy, or by just using your spoon. Transfer to another glass jar, and let finish cooling.

Store in this glass jar with an airtight lid, and keep for up to 6 months.

Scrape Saver

What you will need:

12 drops myrrh oil

8 drops jasmine oil

8 drops tea tree oil

1/3 cup beeswax

½ cup coconut oil

¼ cup shea butter

1/3 cup sweet almond oil

Directions:

Shave the beeswax into a pan on the stove and turn on to medium heat. Add in the coconut oil, and stir as the combination melts.

Continue to stir and keep an eye on the mix, and once it's completely smooth, cut the shea butter into smaller pieces and add that as well. Once the mix is smooth once more, add in the rest of the ingredients.

Remove from heat, and let cool, stirring occasionally. You may need to use your electric mixer to keep it light and fluffy, or by just using your spoon. Transfer to another glass jar, and let finish cooling.

Store in this glass jar with an airtight lid, and keep for up to 6 months.

Angel's Kiss

What you will need:

10 drops cinnamon oil

8 drops vanilla oil

1/3 cup beeswax

½ cup coconut oil

¼ cup shea butter

1/3 cup sweet almond oil

Directions:

Shave the beeswax into a pan on the stove and turn on to medium heat. Add in the coconut oil, and stir as the combination melts.

Continue to stir and keep an eye on the mix, and once it's completely smooth, cut the shea butter into smaller pieces and add that as well. Once the mix is smooth once more, add in the rest of the ingredients.

Remove from heat, and let cool, stirring occasionally. You may need to use your electric mixer to keep it light and fluffy, or by just using your spoon. Transfer to another glass jar, and let finish cooling.

Store in this glass jar with an airtight lid, and keep for up to 6 months.

Cracked Concealer
What you will need:

12 drops myrrh oil

1 teaspoon witch hazel

1/3 cup beeswax

½ cup coconut oil

¼ cup shea butter

1/3 cup sweet almond oil

Directions:

Shave the beeswax into a pan on the stove and turn on to medium heat. Add in the coconut oil, and stir as the combination melts.

Continue to stir and keep an eye on the mix, and once it's completely smooth, cut the shea butter into smaller pieces and add that as well. Once the mix is smooth once more, add in the rest of the ingredients.

Remove from heat, and let cool, stirring occasionally. You may need to use your electric mixer to keep it light and fluffy, or by just using your spoon. Transfer to another glass jar, and let finish cooling.

Store in this glass jar with an airtight lid, and keep for up to 6 months.

Chapter 3 – Salves the Day

Sweetly Scented Savor
What you will need:

1 teaspoon aloe vera juice

10 drops chamomile leaves, crushed

1/3 cup beeswax

½ cup coconut oil

¼ cup shea butter

1/3 cup sweet almond oil

Directions:

Shave the beeswax into a pan on the stove and turn on to medium heat. Add in the coconut oil, and stir as the combination melts.

Continue to stir and keep an eye on the mix, and once it's completely smooth, cut the shea butter into smaller pieces and add that as well. Once the mix is smooth once more, add in the rest of the ingredients.

Remove from heat, and let cool, stirring occasionally. You may need to use your electric mixer to keep it light and fluffy, or by just using your spoon. Transfer to another glass jar, and let finish cooling.

Store in this glass jar with an airtight lid, and keep for up to 6 months.

Happy Salve
What you will need:

12 drops tea tree oil

8 drops geranium oil

1 capsule cod liver oil (make sure this melts completely)

1/3 cup beeswax

½ cup coconut oil

¼ cup shea butter

1/3 cup sweet almond oil

Directions:

Shave the beeswax into a pan on the stove and turn on to medium heat. Add in the coconut oil, and stir as the combination melts.

Continue to stir and keep an eye on the mix, and once it's completely smooth, cut the shea butter into smaller pieces and add that as well. Once the mix is smooth once more, add in the rest of the ingredients.

Remove from heat, and let cool, stirring occasionally. You may need to use your electric mixer to keep it light and fluffy, or by just using your spoon. Transfer to another glass jar, and let finish cooling.

Store in this glass jar with an airtight lid, and keep for up to 6 months.

Soft as Silk
What you will need:

12 drops lavender oil

8 drops lemon oil

1/3 cup beeswax

½ cup coconut oil

¼ cup shea butter

1/3 cup sweet almond oil

Directions:

Shave the beeswax into a pan on the stove and turn on to medium heat. Add in the coconut oil, and stir as the combination melts.

Continue to stir and keep an eye on the mix, and once it's completely smooth, cut the shea butter into smaller pieces and add that as well. Once the mix is smooth once more, add in the rest of the ingredients.

Remove from heat, and let cool, stirring occasionally. You may need to use your electric mixer to keep it light and fluffy, or by just using your spoon. Transfer to another glass jar, and let finish cooling.

Store in this glass jar with an airtight lid, and keep for up to 6 months.

Wintersoft

What you will need:

8 drops lavender oil

8 drops peppermint oil

1 teaspoon aloe vera juice

1/3 cup beeswax

½ cup coconut oil

¼ cup shea butter

1/3 cup sweet almond oil

Directions:

Shave the beeswax into a pan on the stove and turn on to medium heat. Add in the coconut oil, and stir as the combination melts.

Continue to stir and keep an eye on the mix, and once it's completely smooth, cut the shea butter into smaller pieces and add that as well. Once the mix is smooth once more, add in the rest of the ingredients.

Remove from heat, and let cool, stirring occasionally. You may need to use your electric mixer to keep it light and fluffy, or by just using your spoon. Transfer to another glass jar, and let finish cooling.

Store in this glass jar with an airtight lid, and keep for up to 6 months.

Smiles and Sunshine
What you will need:

10 drops lemon oil

8 drops cedar oil

1/3 cup beeswax

½ cup coconut oil

¼ cup shea butter

1/3 cup sweet almond oil

Directions:

Shave the beeswax into a pan on the stove and turn on to medium heat. Add in the coconut oil, and stir as the combination melts.

Continue to stir and keep an eye on the mix, and once it's completely smooth, cut the shea butter into smaller pieces and add that as well. Once the mix is smooth once more, add in the rest of the ingredients.

Remove from heat, and let cool, stirring occasionally. You may need to use your electric mixer to keep it light and fluffy, or by just using your spoon. Transfer to another glass jar, and let finish cooling.

Store in this glass jar with an airtight lid, and keep for up to 6 months.

Chapter 4 – Special Salves for Special Occasions

This is the Salve
What you will need:

1 teaspoon crushed lavender leaves

1 teaspoon crushed green tea leaves

1/3 cup beeswax

½ cup coconut oil

¼ cup shea butter

1/3 cup sweet almond oil

Directions:

Shave the beeswax into a pan on the stove and turn on to medium heat. Add in the coconut oil, and stir as the combination melts.

Continue to stir and keep an eye on the mix, and once it's completely smooth, cut the shea butter into smaller pieces and add that as well. Once the mix is smooth once more, add in the rest of the ingredients.

Remove from heat, and let cool, stirring occasionally. You may need to use your electric mixer to keep it light and fluffy, or by just using your spoon. Transfer to another glass jar, and let finish cooling.

Store in this glass jar with an airtight lid, and keep for up to 6 months.

Super Salve
What you will need:

1 teaspoon witch hazel

8 drops geranium oil

1/3 cup beeswax

½ cup coconut oil

¼ cup shea butter

1/3 cup sweet almond oil

Directions:

Shave the beeswax into a pan on the stove and turn on to medium heat. Add in the coconut oil, and stir as the combination melts.

Continue to stir and keep an eye on the mix, and once it's completely smooth, cut the shea butter into smaller pieces and add that as well. Once the mix is smooth once more, add in the rest of the ingredients.

Remove from heat, and let cool, stirring occasionally. You may need to use your electric mixer to keep it light and fluffy, or by just using your spoon. Transfer to another glass jar, and let finish cooling.

Store in this glass jar with an airtight lid, and keep for up to 6 months.

His or Hers Salve
What you will need:

12 drops cinnamon oil

8 drops clary sage oil

1/3 cup beeswax

½ cup coconut oil

¼ cup shea butter

1/3 cup sweet almond oil

Directions:

Shave the beeswax into a pan on the stove and turn on to medium heat. Add in the coconut oil, and stir as the combination melts.

Continue to stir and keep an eye on the mix, and once it's completely smooth, cut the shea butter into smaller pieces and add that as well. Once the mix is smooth once more, add in the rest of the ingredients.

Remove from heat, and let cool, stirring occasionally. You may need to use your electric mixer to keep it light and fluffy, or by just using your spoon. Transfer to another glass jar, and let finish cooling.

Store in this glass jar with an airtight lid, and keep for up to 6 months.

Just Salves the Day

What you will need:

10 drops ylang ylang oil

6 drops jasmine oil

1/3 cup beeswax

½ cup coconut oil

¼ cup shea butter

1/3 cup sweet almond oil

Directions:

Shave the beeswax into a pan on the stove and turn on to medium heat. Add in the coconut oil, and stir as the combination melts.

Continue to stir and keep an eye on the mix, and once it's completely smooth, cut

the shea butter into smaller pieces and add that as well. Once the mix is smooth once more, add in the rest of the ingredients.

Remove from heat, and let cool, stirring occasionally. You may need to use your electric mixer to keep it light and fluffy, or by just using your spoon. Transfer to another glass jar, and let finish cooling.

Store in this glass jar with an airtight lid, and keep for up to 6 months.

Mom's Favorite Salve
What you will need:

9 drops clary sage oil

8 drops tea tree oil

½ teaspoon witch hazel

1/3 cup beeswax

½ cup coconut oil

¼ cup shea butter

1/3 cup sweet almond oil

Directions:

Shave the beeswax into a pan on the stove and turn on to medium heat. Add in the coconut oil, and stir as the combination melts.

Continue to stir and keep an eye on the mix, and once it's completely smooth, cut the shea butter into smaller pieces and add that as well. Once the mix is smooth once more, add in the rest of the ingredients.

Remove from heat, and let cool, stirring occasionally. You may need to use your electric mixer to keep it light and fluffy, or by just using your spoon. Transfer to another glass jar, and let finish cooling.

Store in this glass jar with an airtight lid, and keep for up to 6 months.

Chapter 5 – A Salve for Everyone

The Sting Eraser

What you will need:

1 teaspoon aloe vera juice

1 teaspoon aloe vera gel

1 teaspoon honey

1/3 cup beeswax

½ cup coconut oil

¼ cup shea butter

1/3 cup sweet almond oil

Directions:

Shave the beeswax into a pan on the stove and turn on to medium heat. Add in the coconut oil, and stir as the combination melts.

Continue to stir and keep an eye on the mix, and once it's completely smooth, cut the shea butter into smaller pieces and add that as well. Once the mix is smooth once more, add in the rest of the ingredients.

Remove from heat, and let cool, stirring occasionally. You may need to use your electric mixer to keep it light and fluffy, or by just using your spoon. Transfer to another glass jar, and let finish cooling.

Store in this glass jar with an airtight lid, and keep for up to 6 months.

Your Little Healer
What you will need:

1 teaspoon aloe vera juice

10 drops vetiver oil

1/3 cup beeswax

½ cup coconut oil

¼ cup shea butter

1/3 cup sweet almond oil

Directions:

Shave the beeswax into a pan on the stove and turn on to medium heat. Add in the coconut oil, and stir as the combination melts.

Continue to stir and keep an eye on the mix, and once it's completely smooth, cut the shea butter into smaller pieces and add that as well. Once the mix is smooth once more, add in the rest of the ingredients.

Remove from heat, and let cool, stirring occasionally. You may need to use your electric mixer to keep it light and fluffy, or by just using your spoon. Transfer to another glass jar, and let finish cooling.

Store in this glass jar with an airtight lid, and keep for up to 6 months.

All Better Bash
What you will need:

12 drops jojoba oil

5 drops cardamom oil

1/3 cup beeswax

½ cup coconut oil

¼ cup shea butter

1/3 cup sweet almond oil

Directions:

Shave the beeswax into a pan on the stove and turn on to medium heat. Add in the coconut oil, and stir as the combination melts.

Continue to stir and keep an eye on the mix, and once it's completely smooth, cut the shea butter into smaller pieces and add that as well. Once the mix is smooth once more, add in the rest of the ingredients.

Remove from heat, and let cool, stirring occasionally. You may need to use your electric mixer to keep it light and fluffy, or by just using your spoon. Transfer to another glass jar, and let finish cooling.

Store in this glass jar with an airtight lid, and keep for up to 6 months.

Handy Salve
What you will need:

1 teaspoon green tea leaves, crushed

12 drops myrrh oil

1/3 cup beeswax

½ cup coconut oil

¼ cup shea butter

1/3 cup sweet almond oil

Directions:

Shave the beeswax into a pan on the stove and turn on to medium heat. Add in the coconut oil, and stir as the combination melts.

Continue to stir and keep an eye on the mix, and once it's completely smooth, cut the shea butter into smaller pieces and add that as well. Once the mix is smooth once more, add in the rest of the ingredients.

Remove from heat, and let cool, stirring occasionally. You may need to use your electric mixer to keep it light and fluffy, or by just using your spoon. Transfer to another glass jar, and let finish cooling.

Store in this glass jar with an airtight lid, and keep for up to 6 months.

Pocket Protector

What you will need:

1 teaspoon green tea leaves, crushed

1 teaspoon rosemary leaves, crushed

1/3 cup beeswax

½ cup coconut oil

¼ cup shea butter

1/3 cup sweet almond oil

Directions:

Shave the beeswax into a pan on the stove and turn on to medium heat. Add in the coconut oil, and stir as the combination melts.

Continue to stir and keep an eye on the mix, and once it's completely smooth, cut the shea butter into smaller pieces and add that as well. Once the mix is smooth once more, add in the rest of the ingredients.

Remove from heat, and let cool, stirring occasionally. You may need to use your electric mixer to keep it light and fluffy, or by just using your spoon. Transfer to another glass jar, and let finish cooling.

Store in this glass jar with an airtight lid, and keep for up to 6 months.

Chapter 6 – Best Salves of All

Salve a Blast
What you will need:

10 drops orange oil

12 drops lavender oil

1/3 cup beeswax

½ cup coconut oil

¼ cup shea butter

1/3 cup sweet almond oil

Directions:

Shave the beeswax into a pan on the stove and turn on to medium heat. Add in the coconut oil, and stir as the combination melts.

Continue to stir and keep an eye on the mix, and once it's completely smooth, cut the shea butter into smaller pieces and add that as well. Once the mix is smooth once more, add in the rest of the ingredients.

Remove from heat, and let cool, stirring occasionally. You may need to use your electric mixer to keep it light and fluffy, or by just using your spoon. Transfer to another glass jar, and let finish cooling.

Store in this glass jar with an airtight lid, and keep for up to 6 months.

Cream of the Crop
What you will need:

1 teaspoon honey

1 teaspoon aloe vera gel

12 drops ylang ylang

10 drops jasmine

1/3 cup beeswax

½ cup coconut oil

¼ cup shea butter

1/3 cup sweet almond oil

Directions:

Shave the beeswax into a pan on the stove and turn on to medium heat. Add in the coconut oil, and stir as the combination melts.

Continue to stir and keep an eye on the mix, and once it's completely smooth, cut the shea butter into smaller pieces and add that as well. Once the mix is smooth once more, add in the rest of the ingredients.

Remove from heat, and let cool, stirring occasionally. You may need to use your electric mixer to keep it light and fluffy, or by just using your spoon. Transfer to another glass jar, and let finish cooling.

Store in this glass jar with an airtight lid, and keep for up to 6 months.

Newly Fresh
What you will need:

12 drops lavender oil

8 drops pine oil

1/3 cup beeswax

½ cup coconut oil

¼ cup shea butter

1/3 cup sweet almond oil

Directions:

Shave the beeswax into a pan on the stove and turn on to medium heat. Add in the coconut oil, and stir as the combination melts.

Continue to stir and keep an eye on the mix, and once it's completely smooth, cut the shea butter into smaller pieces and add that as well. Once the mix is smooth once more, add in the rest of the ingredients.

Remove from heat, and let cool, stirring occasionally. You may need to use your electric mixer to keep it light and fluffy, or by just using your spoon. Transfer to another glass jar, and let finish cooling.

Store in this glass jar with an airtight lid, and keep for up to 6 months.

Power Pop

What you will need:

1 teaspoon witch hazel

12 drops frankincense oil

1/3 cup beeswax

½ cup coconut oil

¼ cup shea butter

1/3 cup sweet almond oil

Directions:

Shave the beeswax into a pan on the stove and turn on to medium heat. Add in the coconut oil, and stir as the combination melts.

Continue to stir and keep an eye on the mix, and once it's completely smooth, cut the shea butter into smaller pieces and add that as well. Once the mix is smooth once more, add in the rest of the ingredients.

Remove from heat, and let cool, stirring occasionally. You may need to use your electric mixer to keep it light and fluffy, or by just using your spoon. Transfer to another glass jar, and let finish cooling.

Store in this glass jar with an airtight lid, and keep for up to 6 months.

What You Asked For
What you will need:

12 drops rose oil

12 drops rosemary oil

1 teaspoon crushed rosemary leaves

1/3 cup beeswax

½ cup coconut oil

¼ cup shea butter

1/3 cup sweet almond oil

Directions:

Shave the beeswax into a pan on the stove and turn on to medium heat. Add in the coconut oil, and stir as the combination melts.

Continue to stir and keep an eye on the mix, and once it's completely smooth, cut the shea butter into smaller pieces and add that as well. Once the mix is smooth once more, add in the rest of the ingredients.

Remove from heat, and let cool, stirring occasionally. You may need to use your electric mixer to keep it light and fluffy, or by just using your spoon. Transfer to another glass jar, and let finish cooling.

Store in this glass jar with an airtight lid, and keep for up to 6 months.

Conclusion

There you have it, everything you need to know to make your own healing salves, for a variety of uses. I know it's hard to always choose store bought remedies, especially when you aren't sure of what they put into all of them.

But, when you make your own, you have full confidence of what is going into each and every one, and know without a doubt that you are getting the product you want.

Let this book inspire you, and don't just make the salves you find here, but go on and make even more. Mix and match to get what you want, every time.

You are a wizard, so own it!

FREE Bonus Reminder

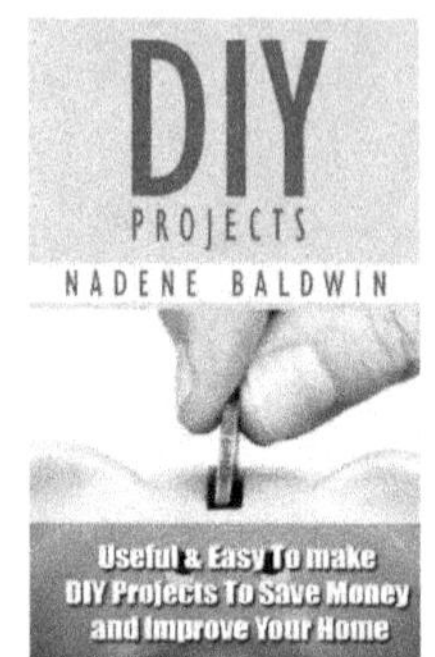

If you have not grabbed it yet, please go ahead and download your special bonus report *"DIY Projects. 13 Useful & Easy To Make DIY Projects To Save Money & Improve Your Home!"*
Simply Click the Button Below

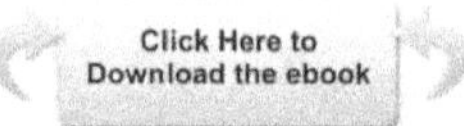

OR **Go to This Page**
http://diyhomecraft.com/free

BONUS #2: More Free & Discounted Books or Products
Do you want to receive more Free/Discounted Books or Products?
We have a mailing list where we send out our new Books or Products when they go free or with a discount on Amazon. Click on the link below to sign up for Free & Discount Book & Product Promotions.
=> Sign Up for Free & Discount Book & Product Promotions <=

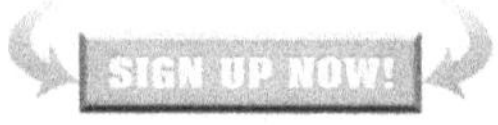

OR Go to this URL
http://zbit.ly/1WBb1Ek

www.ingramcontent.com/pod-product-compliance
Lightning Source LLC
Chambersburg PA
CBHW060822260726
48660CB00003B/1048